MEDICAL ASSISTANT COLORING BOOK

THIS BOOK BELONGS TO

_____

Published by Gahrelukarkhana Publishing

COLOR TEST PAGE

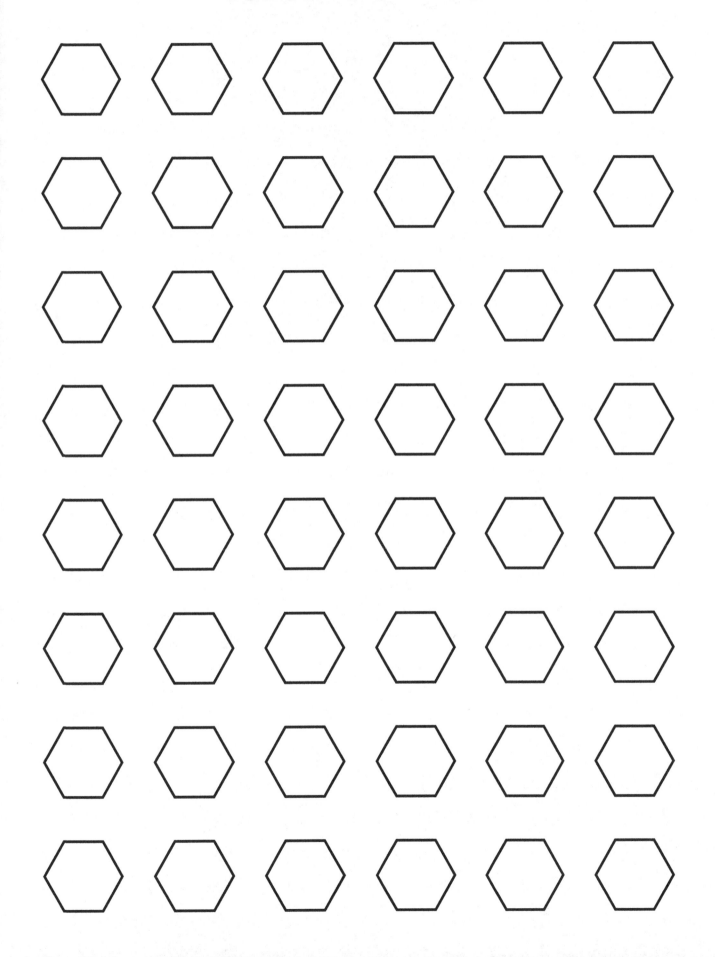

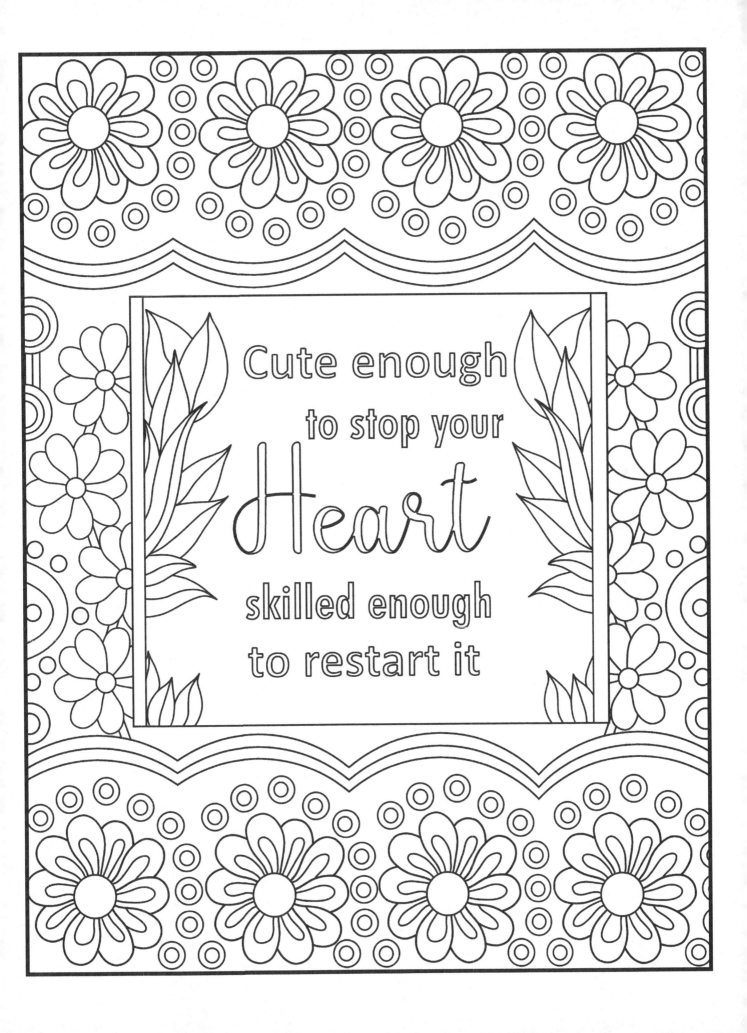

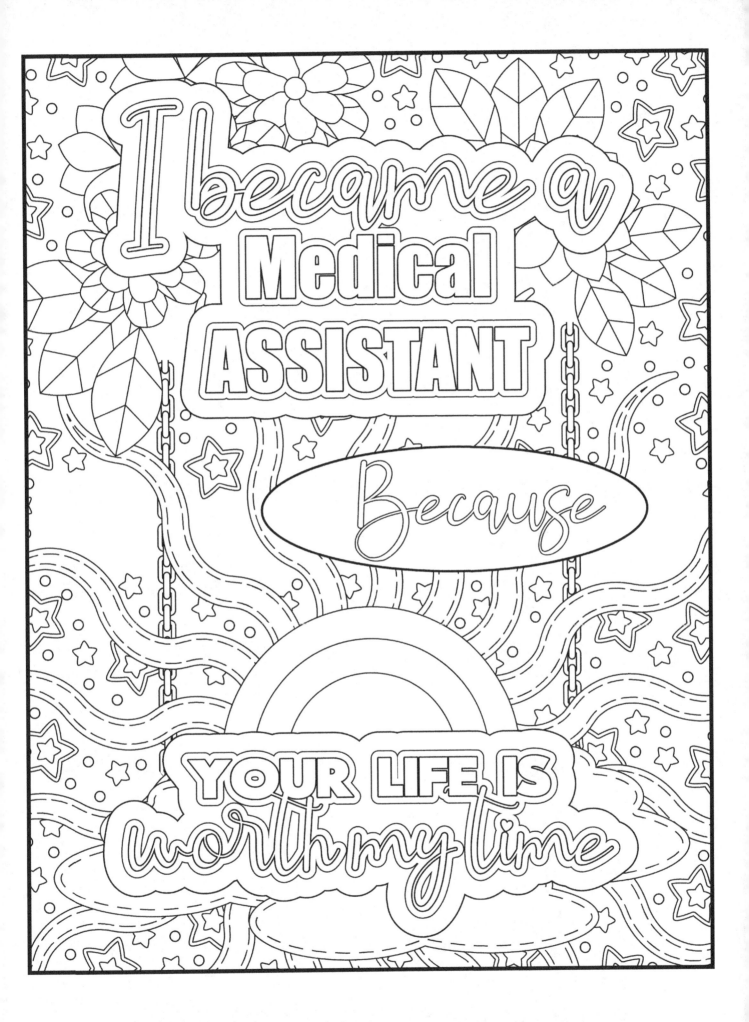

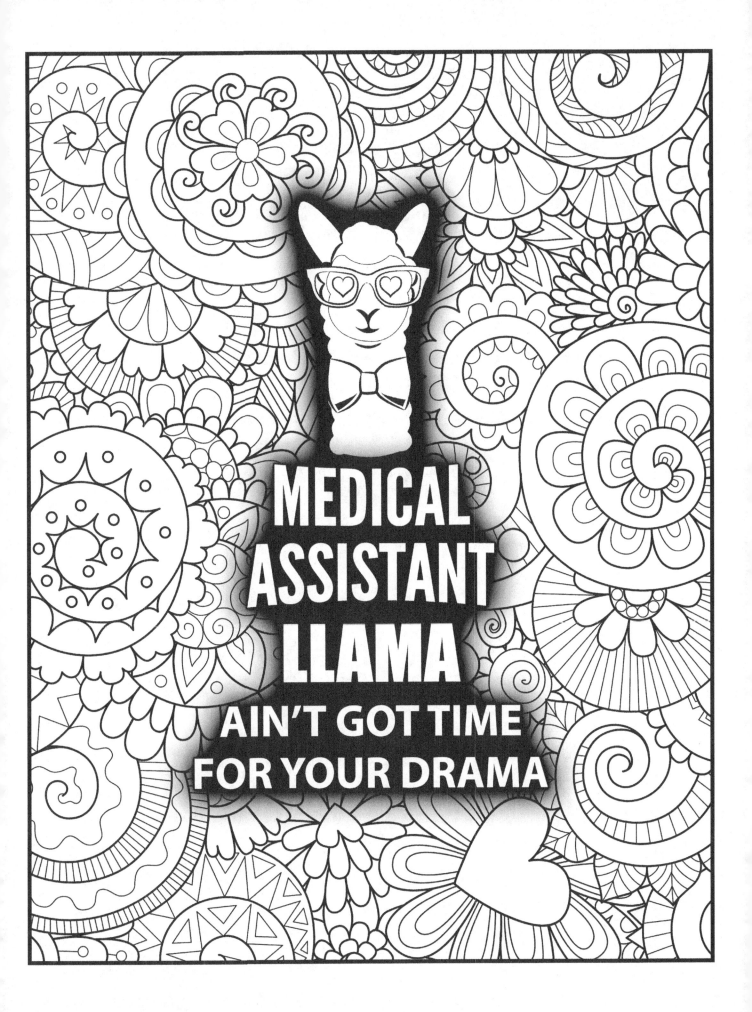

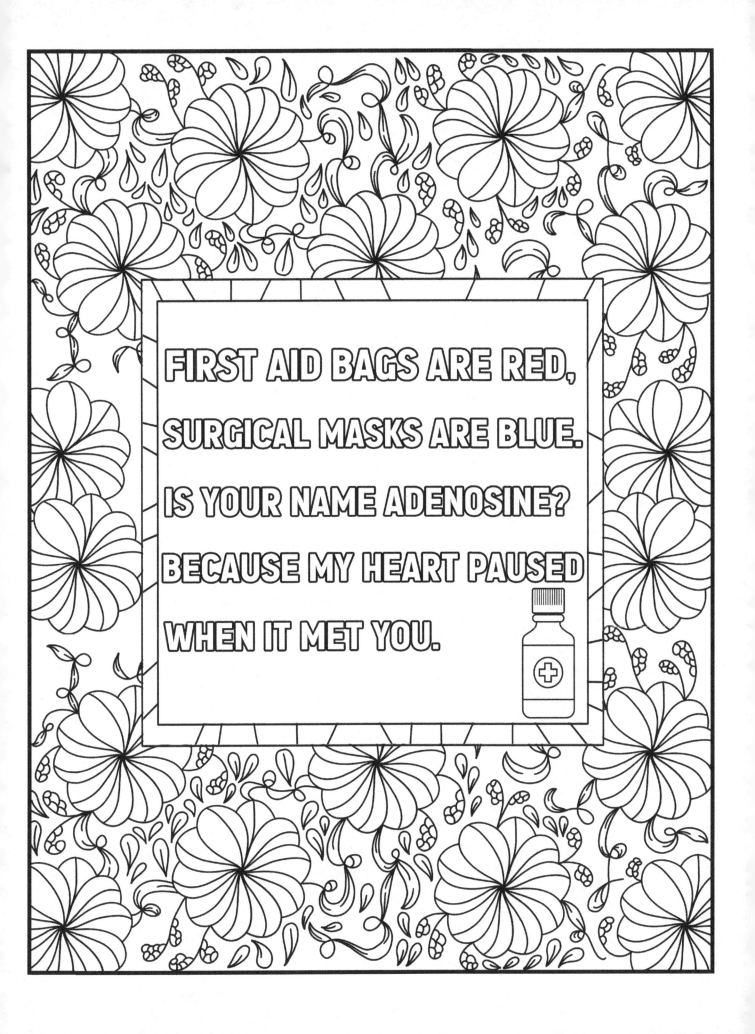

FIRST AID BAGS ARE RED, SURGICAL MASKS ARE BLUE. IS YOUR NAME ADENOSINE? BECAUSE MY HEART PAUSED WHEN IT MET YOU.

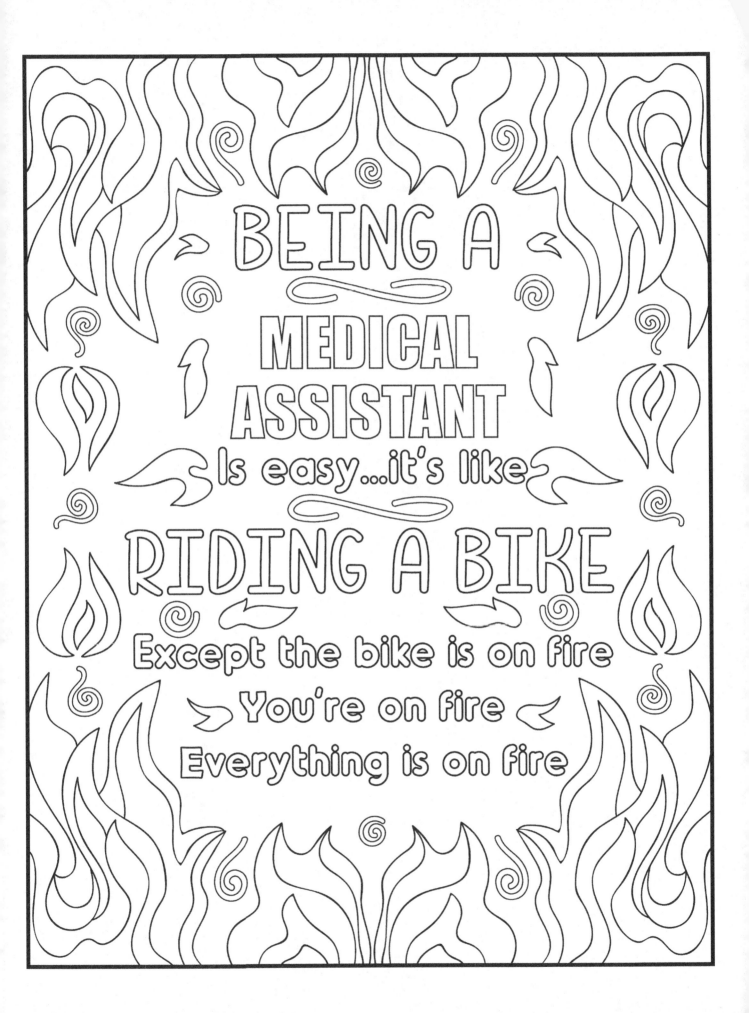

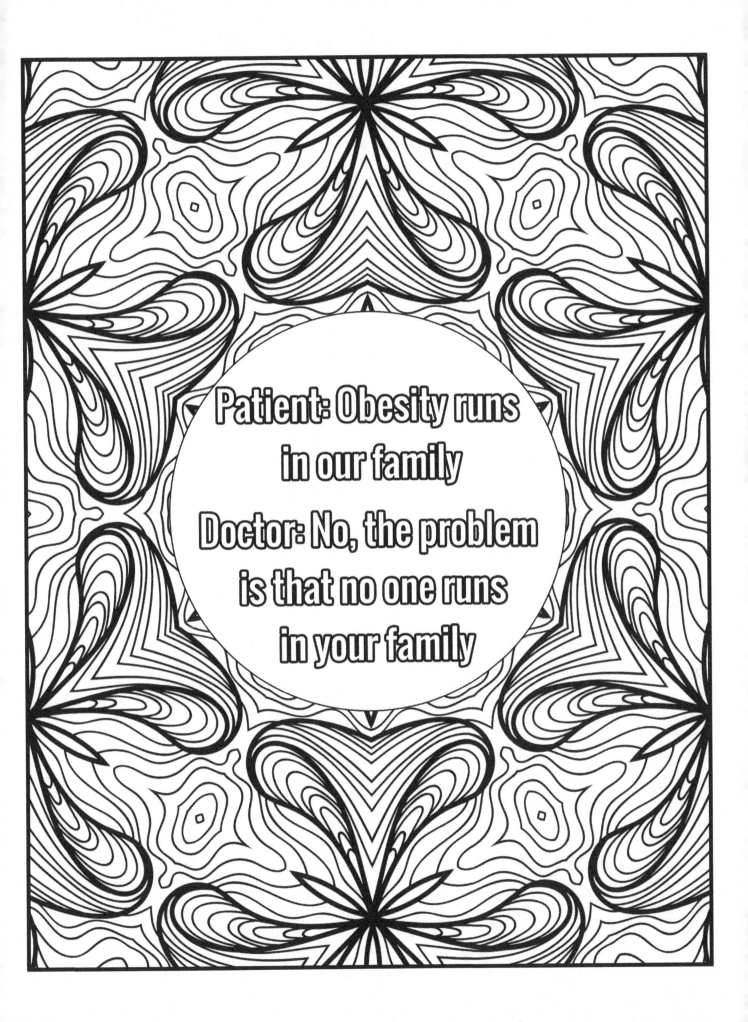

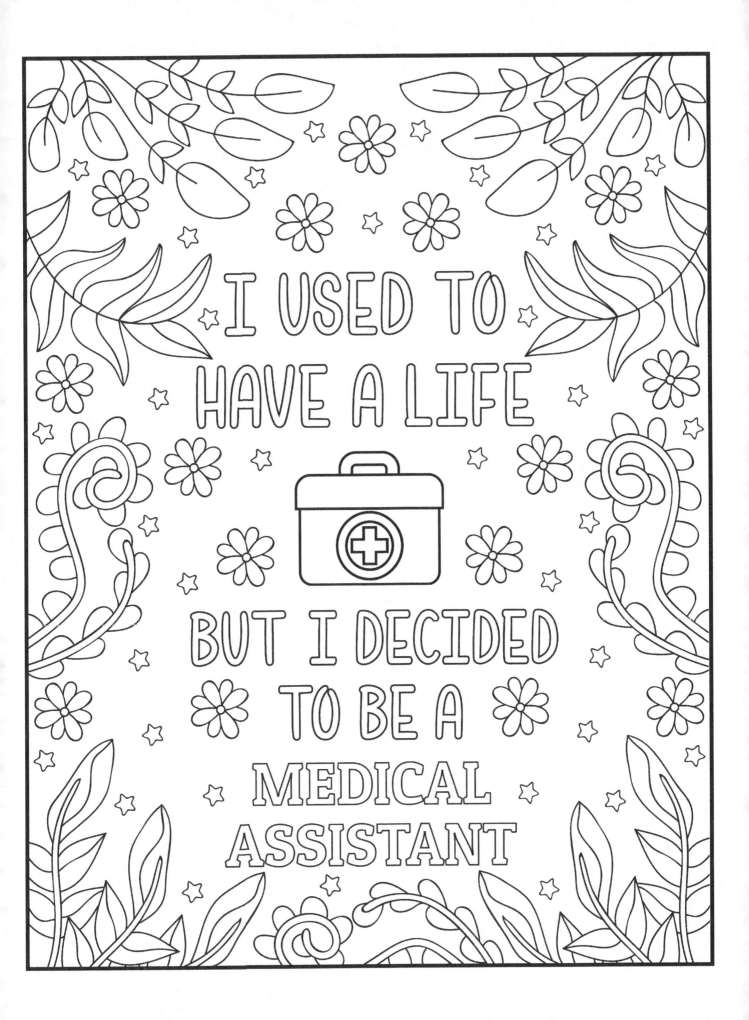

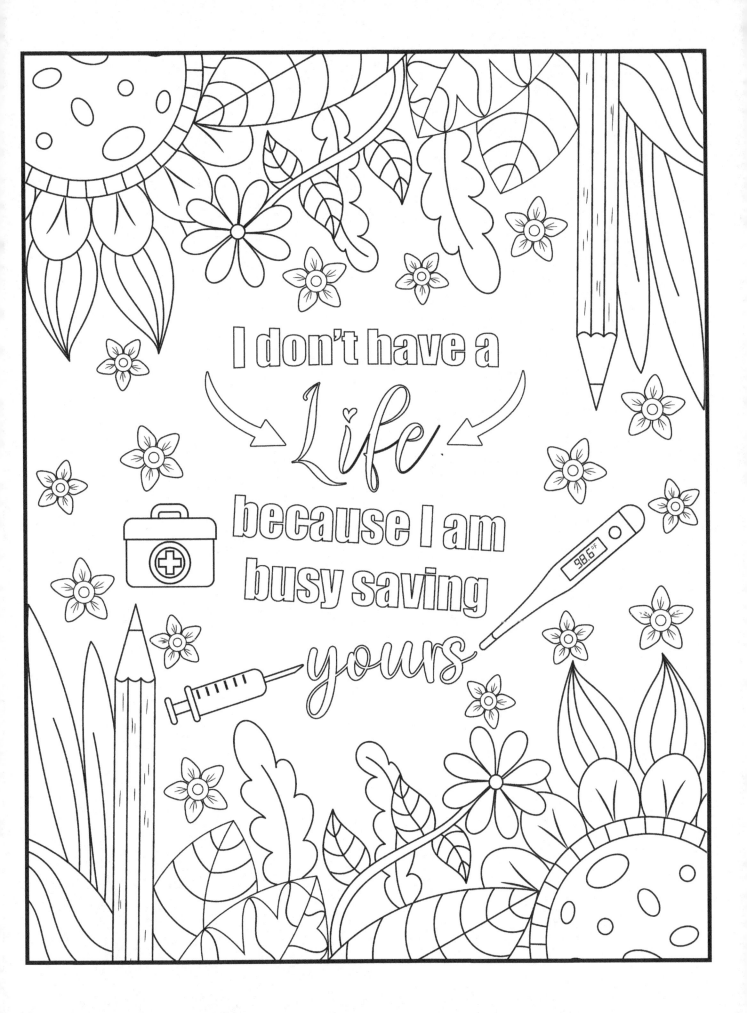

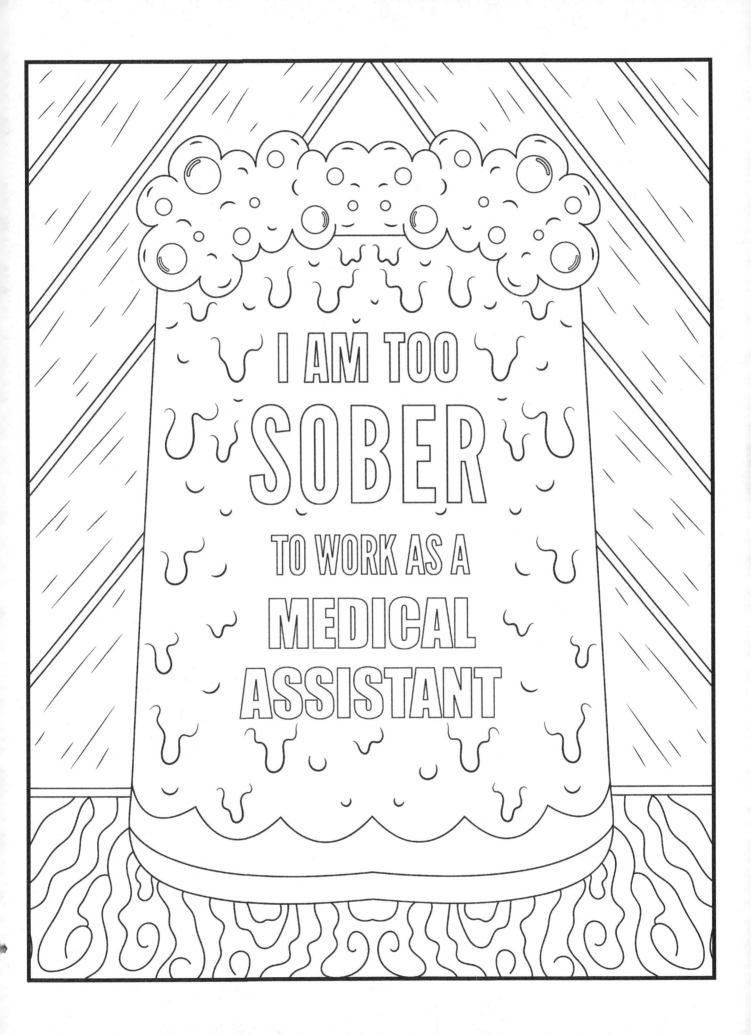

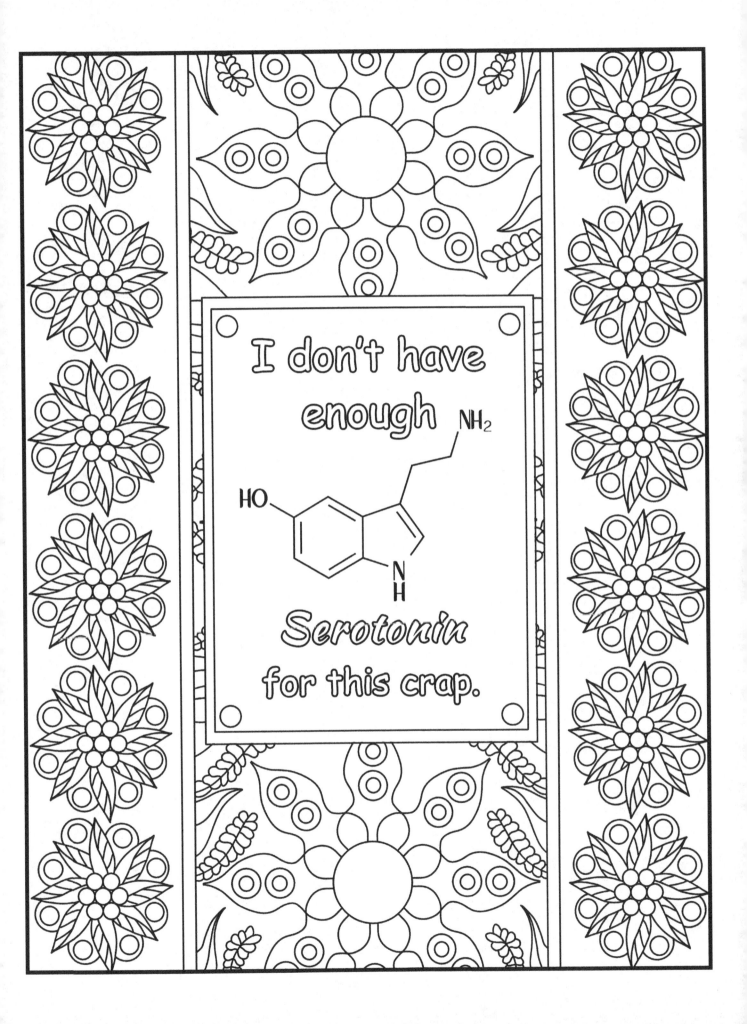

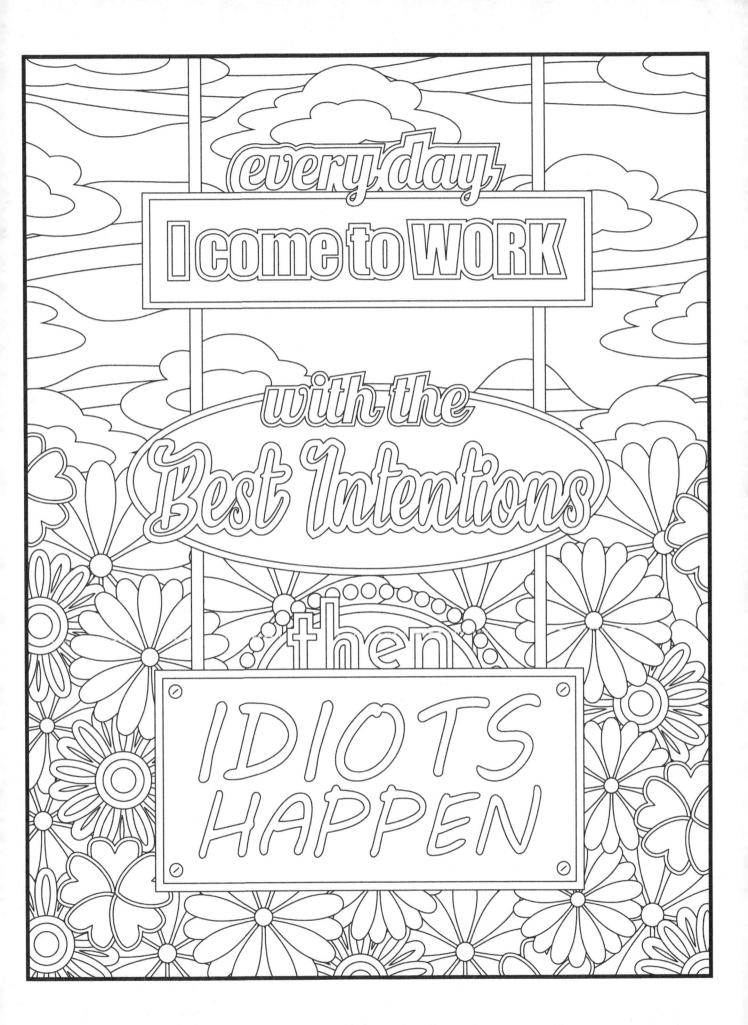

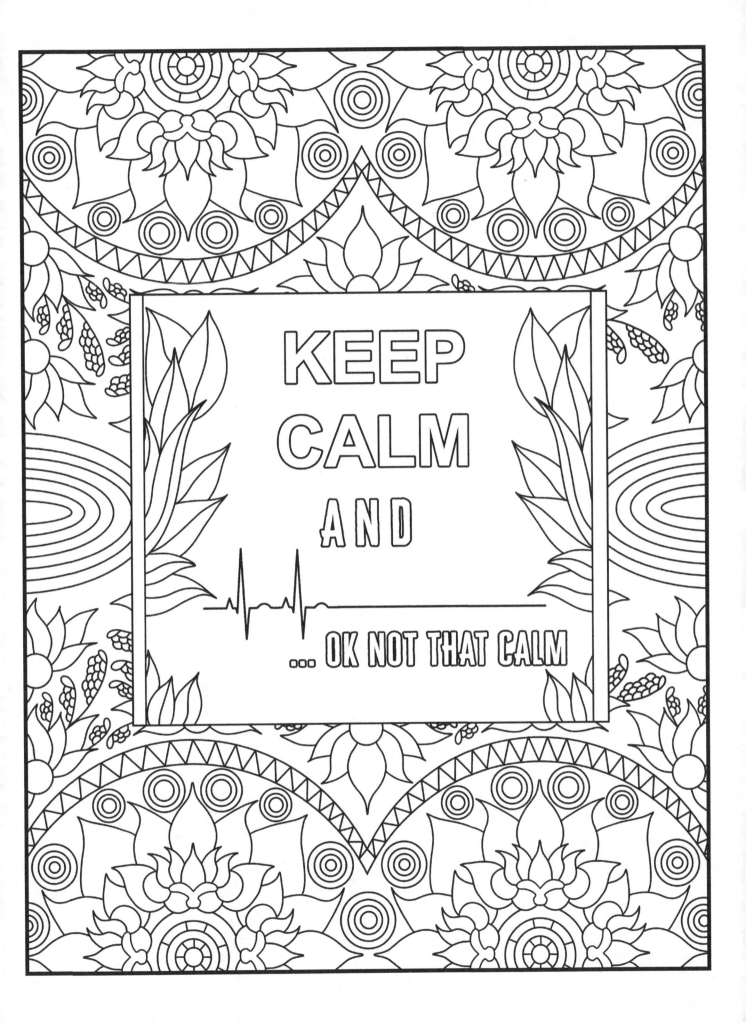

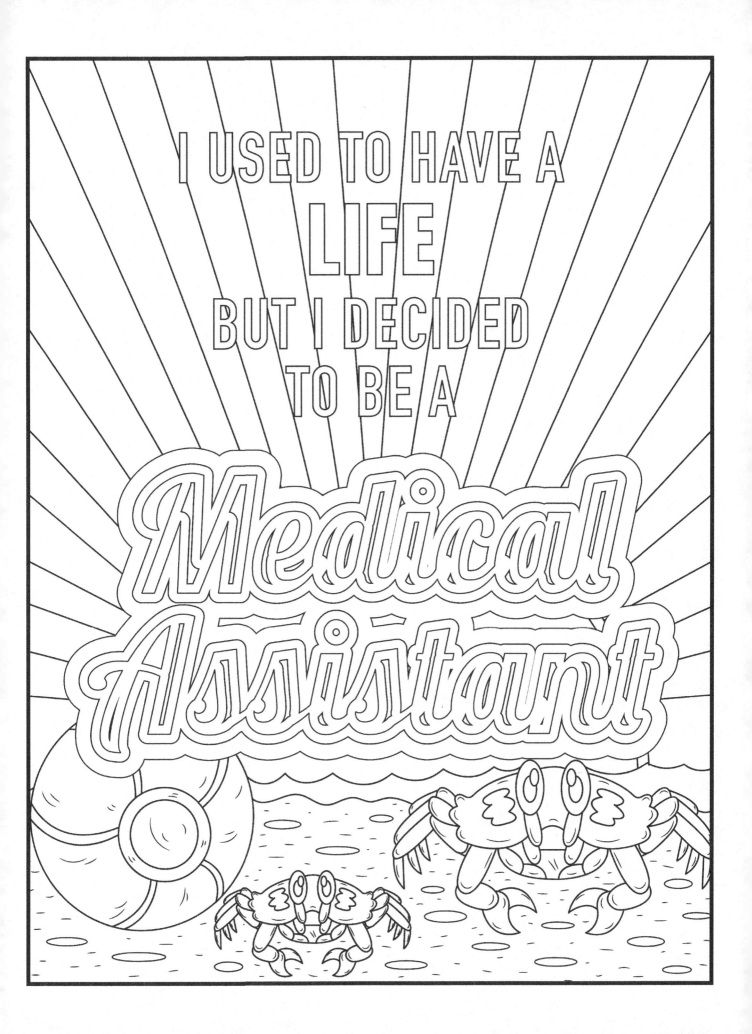

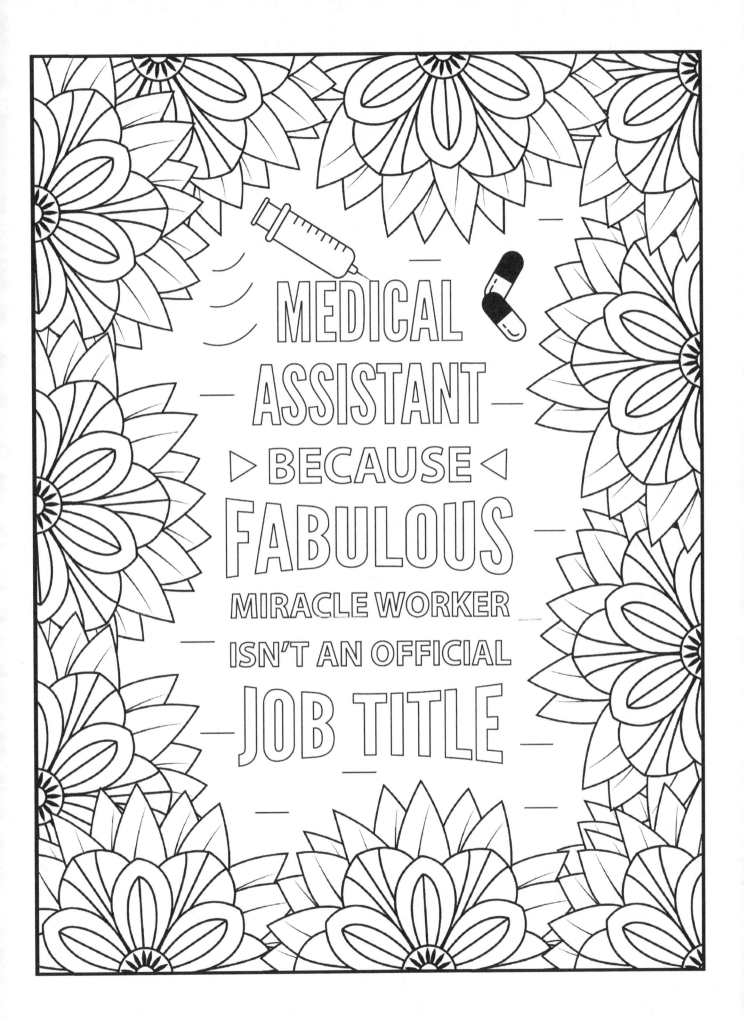

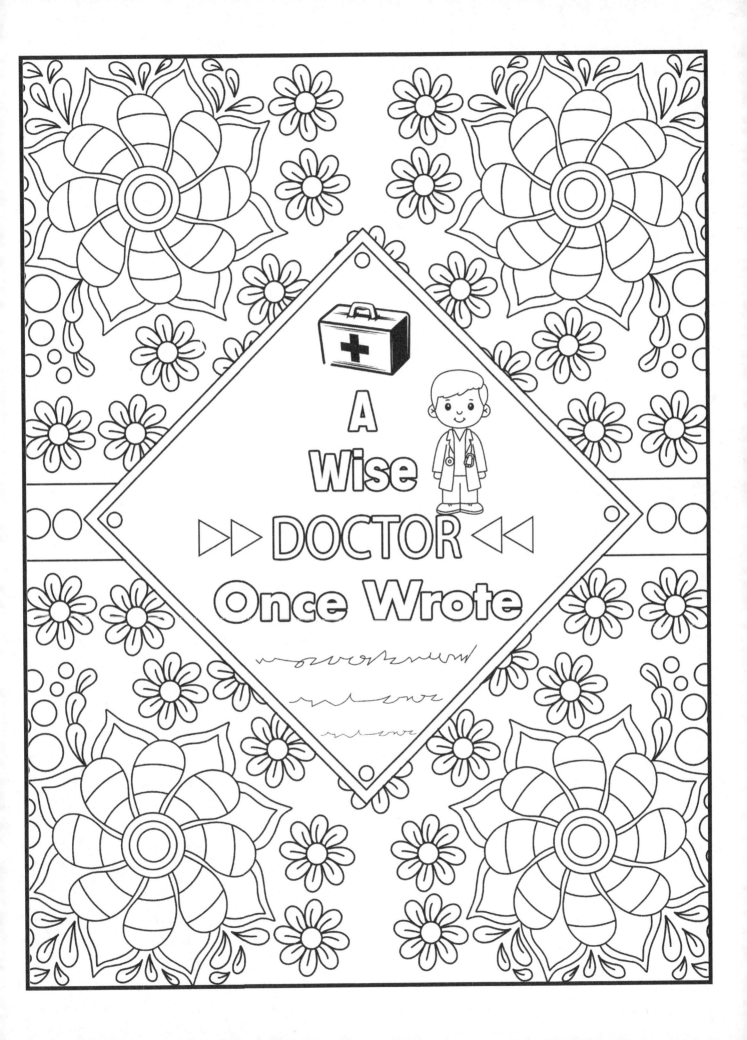

A Wise ▷▷ DOCTOR ◁◁ Once Wrote

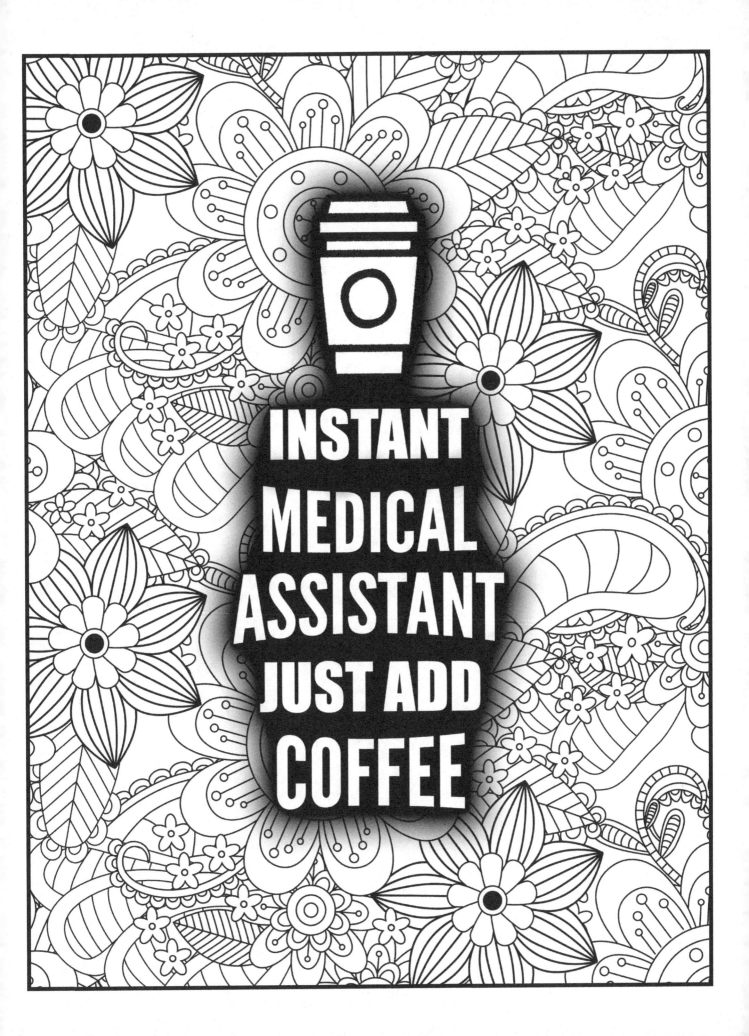

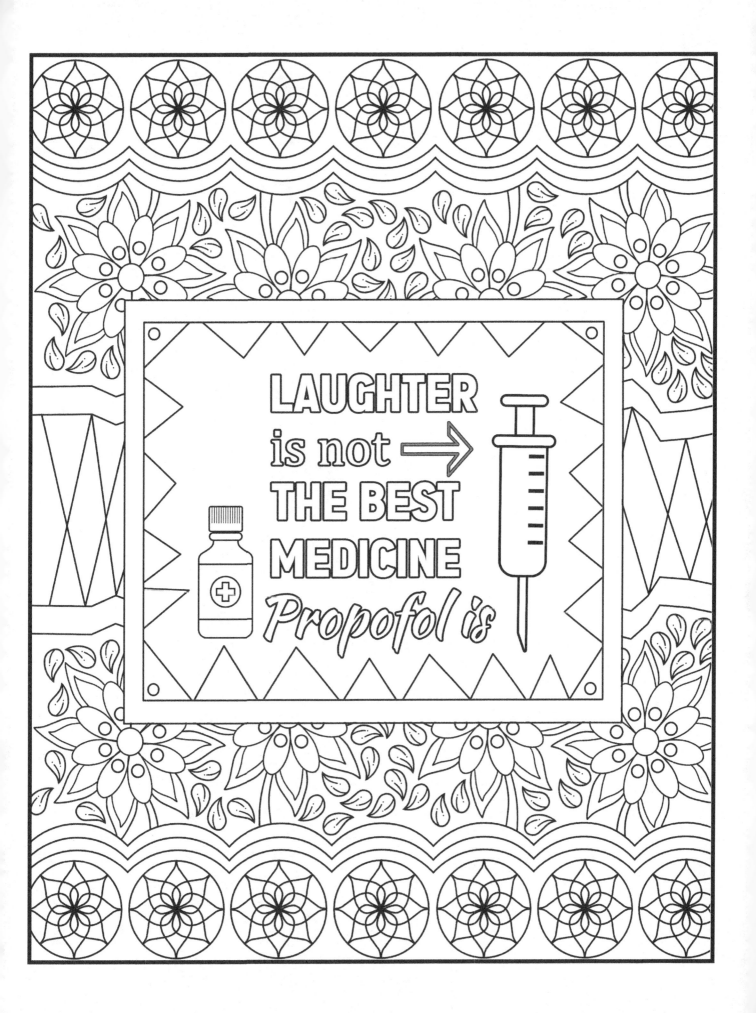

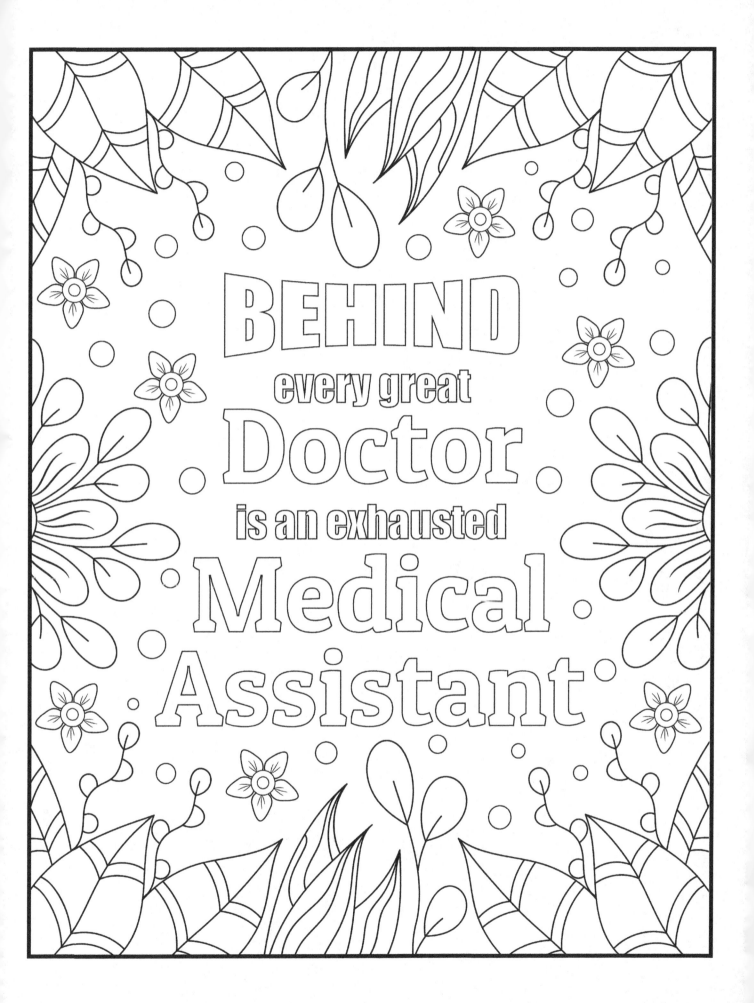

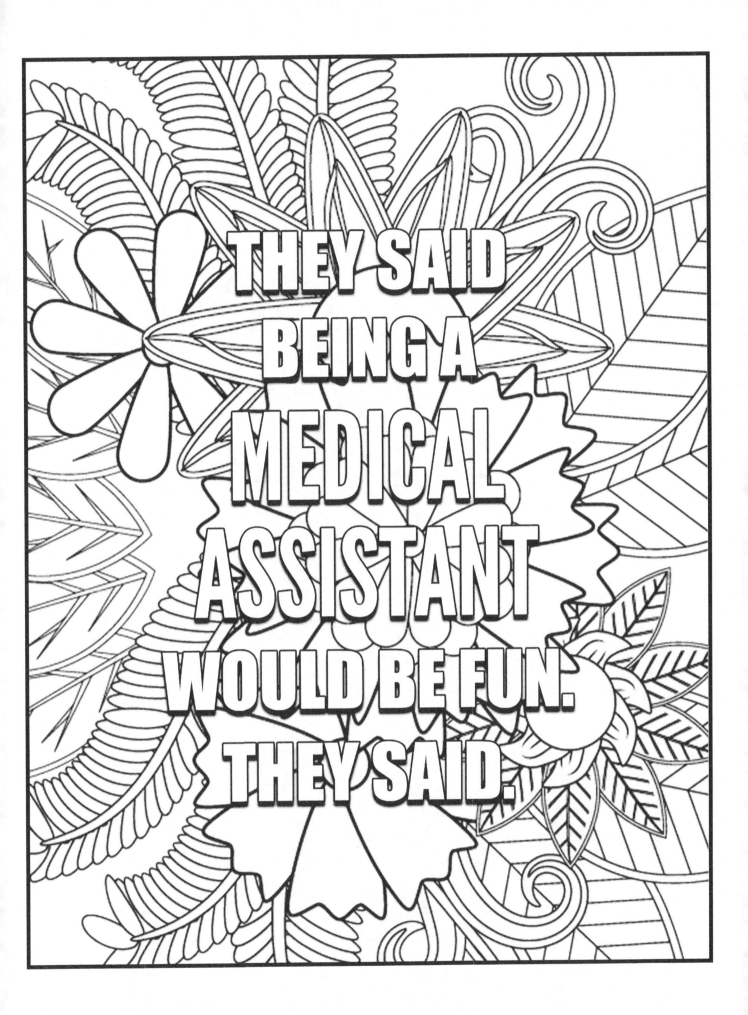

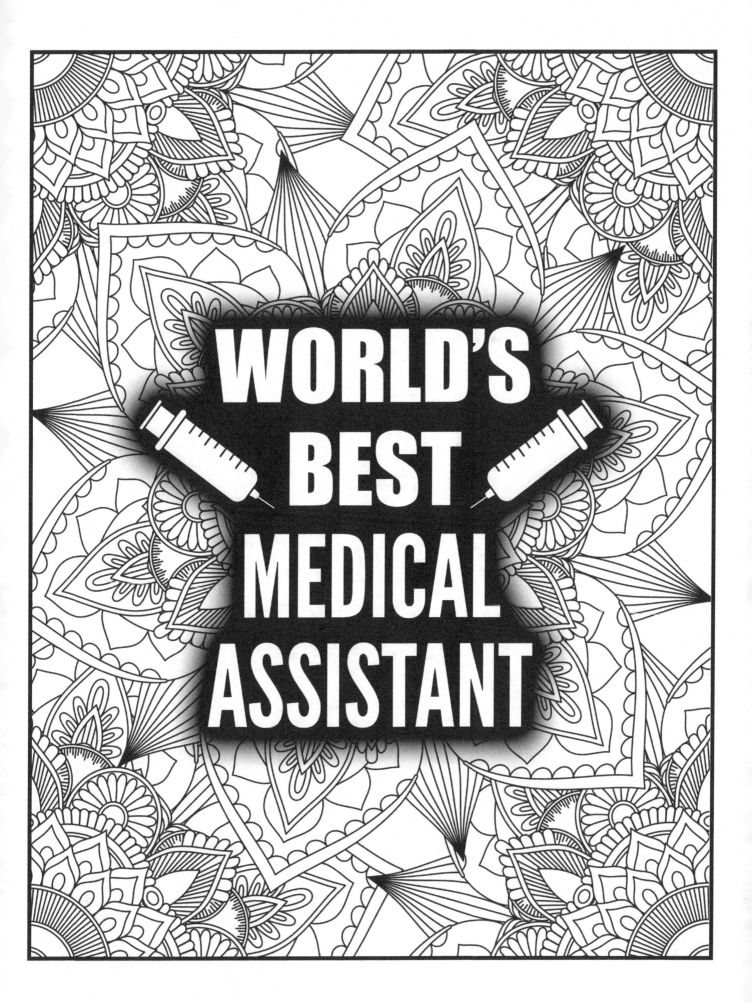

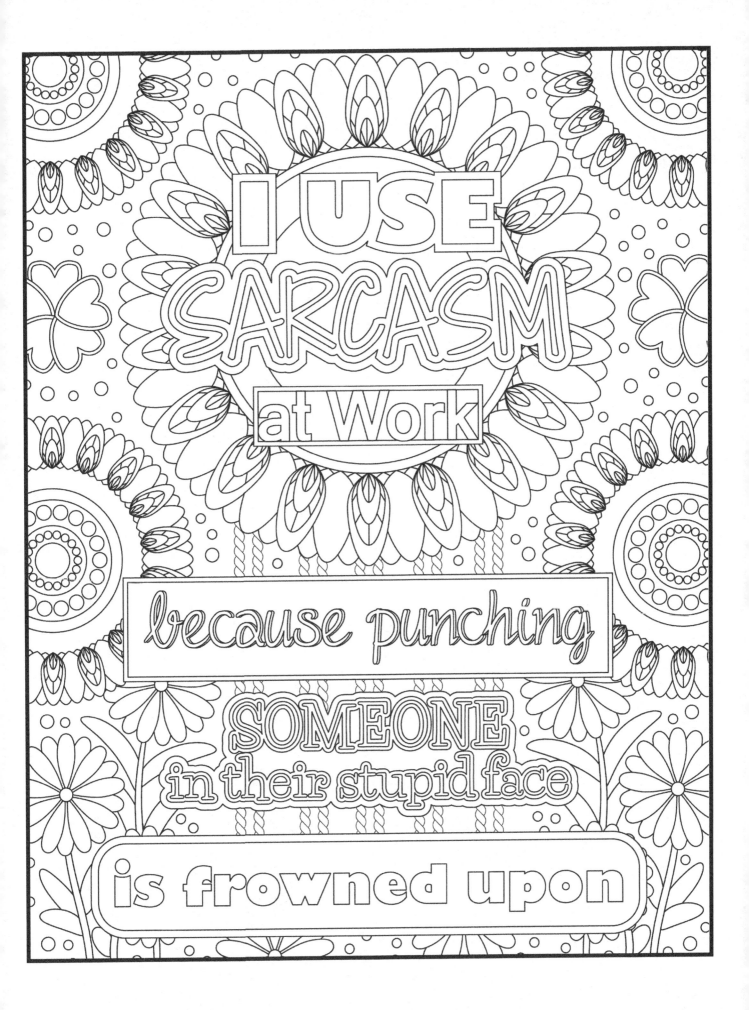

Made in the USA
Las Vegas, NV
01 November 2023

80023680R00026